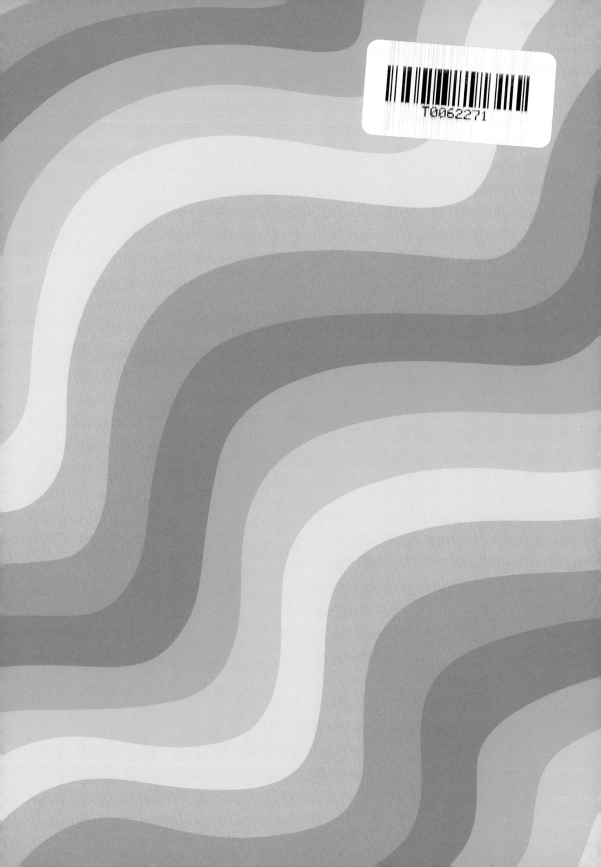

THE QUEER-IODIC TABLE

(ACE EDITION)

1 **W** World domination									2 **R** Sex repulsed aces
3 **Ga** Garlic bread	4 **O** Outer space					5 **Ob** Oblivious aces	6 **Ad** Sex averse aces
7 **C** Cake	8 **Dr** Dragons	9 **A** Asexual	10 **D** Demisexual	11 **V** Valid	12 **Oo** Oodles of validity	13 **In** Innuendo aces	14 **N** Sex neutral aces
15 **Bl** Black ring	16 **Ev** Everything purple	17 **Ac** Aceflux	18 **Gs** Greysexual	19 **Vc** Valid concentrate	20 **S** Super valid	21 **Ro** Alloromantic aces	22 **F** Sex favourable aces
23 **Ax** Axolotls	24 **Sp** Ace of spades	25 **No** Not broken	26 **G** Grey spectrum identities	27 **Va** Valid absolute	28 **H** Hetero-romantic aces	29 **Ar** Aromantic aces	30 **Hi** High libido aces

COMMUNITY   ASEXUALITY   PRIDE   DIVERSITY

AMAZING ACE, AWESOME ARO

of related interest

Perfectly Queer
An Illustrated Introduction
Victoria Barron
ISBN 978 1 83997 714 5
eISBN 978 1 83997 715 2

Hopeless Aromantic
An Affirmative Guide to Aromanticism
Samantha Rendle
ISBN 978 1 83997 367 3
eISBN 978 1 83997 368 0

I Am Ace
Advice on Living Your Best Asexual Life
Cody Daigle-Orians
ISBN 978 1 83997 262 1
eISBN 978 1 83997 263 8

Ace Notes
Tips and Tricks on Existing in an Allo World
Michele Kirichanskaya
Illustrated by Ashley Masog
ISBN 978 1 83997 522 6
eISBN 978 1 83997 523 3

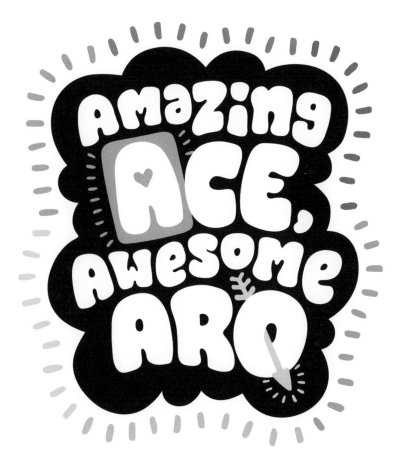

Amazing ACE, Awesome ARO

An Illustrated Exploration

Victoria Barron

Jessica Kingsley Publishers
London and Philadelphia

First published in Great Britain in 2023 by Jessica Kingsley Publishers
An imprint of Hodder & Stoughton Ltd
An Hachette Company

1

Front cover image source: Victoria Barron.

A CIP catalogue record for this title is available from the British Library
and the Library of Congress

ISBN 978 1 83997 714 5
eISBN 978 1 83997 715 2

Printed and bound in China by Leo Paper Products Limited

Jessica Kingsley Publishers' policy is to use papers that are natural,
renewable, and recyclable products and made from wood grown
in sustainable forests. The logging and manufacturing processes
are expected to conform to the environmental regulations
of the country of origin.

Jessica Kingsley Publishers
Carmelite House
50 Victoria Embankment
London EC4Y 0DZ

www.jkp.com

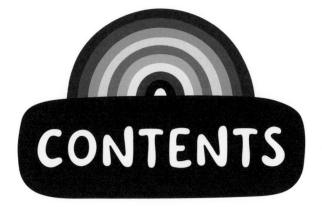

CONTENTS

THE AUTHOR'S STORY

Content warning: *Brief mentions of coerced pressure/behaviour, internalised phobia, self-hate, anxiety, and depression.*

Oh, lovely reader, if only I'd been aware of the asexual and aromantic spectrums earlier in life—I like to think it might have saved myself a lot of confusion and self-hatred in the long run. As it was, my stark awareness of the importance society placed on sexual or romantic attraction (along with my complete lack of awareness about the ace/aro spectrums) resulted in feelings of 'otherness' and 'brokenness', which certainly contributed to my struggles with anxiety, depression, and the negative effects/behaviours I formed to cope.

I'd never really fit the encouraged societal 'norms/standards/expectations', being too loud, too fat, too silly, too unfocused (or randomly hyper-focused); oftentimes feeling easily overwhelmed with emotions, tasks, or sensory input. Even upon my discovery of the ace/aro spectrums, the internalised phobia I experienced came from a place of shame, just one more thing that seemed to confirm how 'different' I was from the expected 'norm'.

In recent years—encouraged through mental health therapy—I've largely been focused on addressing complex trauma and behaviours through education, self-reflection, understanding, and an ongoing reminder that 'different' is inherently neutral—neither good nor bad. And so, while reflecting on the actions of my past, I learnt to distinguish the many forms of attraction I *do* distinctly and consistently experience. I can now recognise that any activity with another person—that would, for most others, be motivated by sexual/romantic attraction—was never because *I personally* experienced that distinct and consistent feeling/desire...only a societal/peer pressure to think/act/behave as was expected of me.

Educating myself and connecting with LGBTQ+ communities provided a major lifeline; where the expectations and pressures of an 'allocishet' society felt excluding and oppressive, the queer connections and support I found provided a sense of place and acceptance. Finally, things made sense. I wasn't 'broken'; I just experienced things in a way that was different...and that was okay.

My personal experience of attraction—how it's experienced and the multiple genders I experience it towards—still feels pretty varied and complex...yet, I finally feel comfortable with my identity. Mine is but one experience, and it can highlight the diversity not only of the spectrums, but the way(s) it can be experienced.

So, whatever your (metaphorical) orientation b-**aro**-meter indicates, I hope you can learn to embr-**ace** your identity knowing that you're not alone!

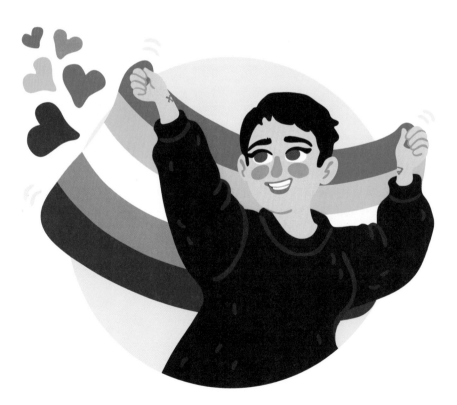

ABOUT THE BOOK

Following the broader focus of LGBTQ+ identities within *Perfectly Queer: An Illustrated Introduction*, the aim of this book is to provide a one-stop resource on the (often misunderstood) area of asexuality and aromanticism. A focus is made on the similarities, yet notable differences, between both the asexual and aromantic spectrums by building an understanding around the orientations from the ground up.

Various nuggets of digestible information combine with engaging illustrations in an effort to provide the tools needed to navigate each section, covering everything from terminology, history, culture, attitudes, split attraction, and much more.

For the amazing ace, the awesome aros, and all the intrigued folks out there, let's explore the wonderful aspects of asexuality and aromanticism!

Disclaimer

Identity flags, terms, and definitions may change/evolve over time and no offence or confusion is intended should any such changes conflict with the contents of this publication. All information was deemed correct at the time of design, with terms and identities combining a variety of factors to create their definitions (including the voices of the acespec and arospec communities, dictionary descriptions, and a personal interpretation/understanding).

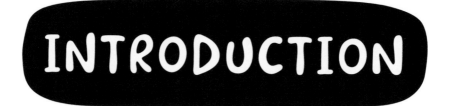

INTRODUCTION

BUILDING AN ACESPEC AND AROSPEC FOUNDATION

This section provides a foundation from which to better recognise how asexuality and aromanticism are defined and distinguished in terms of attraction and orientation.

What do 'ace' and 'aro' mean?

Ace is a label for an individual who has any identity on the *asexual spectrum*.

Aro (pronounced either 'arrow' or 'aye-row') is a label for an individual who has any identity on the *aromantic spectrum*.

'Asexual spectrum' and 'aromantic spectrum'?

The asexual spectrum (commonly shortened to 'acespec') contains a variety of sexual orientations in which little to no *sexual attraction* is experienced.

The aromantic spectrum (commonly shortened to 'arospec') contains a variety of romantic orientations in which little to no *romantic attraction* is experienced.

What are 'sexual attraction' and 'romantic attraction'?

Sexual attraction is a desire to engage in sexual activity (in real life) with a specific person and usually occurs post-puberty (before which a person might experience other *forms of attraction* towards specific genders: romantic, aesthetic, emotional etc.).

Romantic attraction is a desire to engage in a typical/traditional romantic relationship or romantic behaviour (in real life) with a specific person.

What are the different forms of attraction?

The experience of sexual attraction (how, and to whom) is what defines an individual's *sexual orientation*, and the experience of romantic attraction (how, and to whom) is what defines an individual's *romantic orientation*.

Forms of attraction beyond sexual and romantic are often referred to as 'tertiary attraction' (or 'eriattraction'). All forms of attraction (sexual, romantic, and tertiary) may occur simultaneously alongside each other, although tertiary attractions are not specifically used to classify sexual or romantic orientations.

Examples of tertiary attractions include:

- Physical: finding a particular physique or physical trait of a specific person attractive/appealing.

- Sensual: a desire for intimate/bonding touch (sexual or non-sexual) with a specific person.

- Emotional: feeling an emotional connection to the 'inner self' of a person.

- Aesthetic: feeling attracted to the look/style/presentation of a person.

- Platonic: a desire for a close, non-romantic relationship with a person.

- Alterous: a desire for closeness that falls ambiguously between platonic and romantic attraction.

What defines 'sexual orientation' and 'romantic orientation'?

Sexual orientation is often understood as who sexual attraction is experienced towards, but it also includes how sexual attraction is experienced differently to *allosexual* orientations.

Likewise, romantic orientation often concerns who romantic attraction is experienced towards, but also includes how romantic attraction is experienced differently to *alloromantic* orientations.

But what are 'allosexual' and 'alloromantic'?

Allosexuality is at one end of the ace-allo spectrum, whereas the asexual spectrum resides at the other. An allosexual person (whether straight or LGBTQ+) can innately, and distinctly, and consistently experience sexual attraction.

ACE-ALLO SPECTRUM*

ASEXUALITY   **ALLOSEXUALITY**

ASEXUAL SPECTRUM

Acespec orientations that innately experience inconsistent, and/or indistinct sexual attraction, or no sexual attraction whatsoever.

Any sexual orientation (including heterosexual) that innately, consistently, and distinctly experiences sexual attraction.

✱ *NOTE:* fluid/shifting orientations (demi-sexual, lithosexual etc.) can shift anywhere between asexuality and allosexuality.

Alloromanticism is at one end of the aro-allo spectrum, whereas the aromantic spectrum resides at the other. An alloromantic person (whether straight or LGBTQ+) can innately, and distinctly, and consistently experience romantic attraction.

ARO-ALLO SPECTRUM*

AROMANTICISM · **ALLOROMANTICISM**

AROMANTIC SPECTRUM

Arospec orientations that innately experience inconsistent, and/or indistinct romantic attraction, or no romantic attraction whatsoever.

Any romantic orientation (including heteroromantic) that innately, consistently, and distinctly experiences romantic attraction.

✱ *NOTE*: fluid/shifting orientations (demiromantic, lithoromantic etc.) can shift anywhere between aromanticism and allo-romanticism.

Why are asexuality and aromanticism considered LGBTQ+?

Where allosexual and alloromantic orientations can be either straight or queer/LGBTQ+ (dependent on who the attraction is experienced towards), acespec and arospec orientations are only considered to be queer.

Asexuality and aromanticism focus on how little to no sexual attraction is experienced, and for this reason, the ability to experience attraction towards another person will not be innate, and distinct, and consistent. Acespec orientations, therefore, cannot be classified as (or entirely) heterosexual, while arospec orientations, equally, cannot be classified as (or entirely) heteroromantic.

NOTE: A **non-LGBTQ+** individual will be dyadic (i.e. not intersex) *and/or* allocishet (allo-sexual/romantic, *and* cisgender, *and* hetero-sexual/romantic). However, an individual would *(or could, according to preference)* be LGBTQ+ if at least one part of their identity or classification diverges from this list.

For example: a dyadic (non intersex), cisgender man (a man who feels their assigned gender matches their identity), who is asexual (experiences no sexual attraction regardless of gender) and heteroromantic (experiences romantic attraction to a different gender), could identify under the LGBTQ+ umbrella because part of their identity—their sexual orientation—is not allocishet.

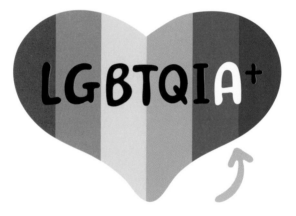

The 'A' commonly stands for acespec, arospec, and agender identities.

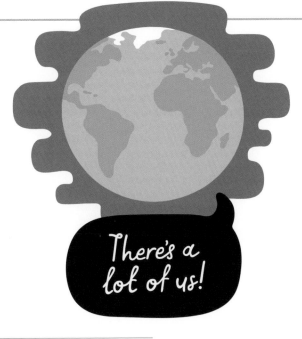

✳ DID YOU KNOW? ✳

Most refer to the survey analysed by Anthony F. Bogaert in 2004[1] that showed 1% (of adults in British households) identifying as asexual. However, within Britain, reports show 5% of people aged 16–26 now identifying as ace,[2] and, with a world population of around 8 billion people,[3] even a 1% estimate creates a possible 8 million acespec people!

No estimates have yet been produced for the numbers of exclusively arospec people, though interestingly the 2020 Ace Community Survey Summary Report records 41.5% of all respondents also identifying as arospec.[4]

There's a lot of us!

1   Bogaert, A.F. (2004) 'Asexuality: Prevalence and associated factors in a national probability sample.' *Journal of Sex Research 41*, 3, 279–287. doi:10.1080/00224490 409552235.

2   Kelly, N. and de Santos, R. (2022) *Rainbow Britain: Attraction, Identity and Connection in Great Britain in 2022*. London: Stonewall. Available at: www.stonewall.org.uk/system/files/rainbow_britain_report.pdf, p.6.

3   According to https://populationmatters.org

4   Hermann, L., Baba, A., Montagner, D., *et al.* (2022) *2020 Ace Community Survey Summary Report*. The Ace Community Survey Team. Available at: https://acecommunitysurvey.org, p.16.

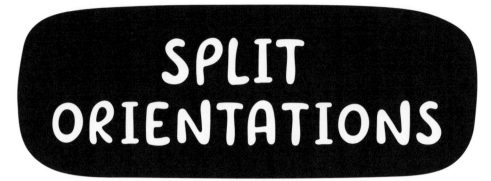

SPLIT ORIENTATIONS

THE SPLIT ATTRACTION MODEL AND VARIORIENTED IDENTITIES

HOW WHAT WHO   WHAT
↓   ↓   ↓   ↓   ↓
greysexual **&** homo-sexual/romantic (e.g. greysexual lesbian)

HOW WHAT   WHO WHAT
↓   ↓   ↓   ↓
demiromantic **&** panromantic (aka: demi-panromantic)

HOW WHAT WHAT HOW
↓   ↓   ↓   ↓
asexual **&** aro**flux**

Decoding identity labels

To better understand how attractions (and therefore orientations) can be distinctly split, it can be useful to 'decode' identity labels. Some labels will provide all relevant information to an individual's sexual and romantic orientation, while others will only state partial aspects. Sections of an identity label can be divided into three possible categories:

- *Who* attraction is experienced towards (using prefixes such as: pan, bi, omni etc.).

- *How* attraction is experienced (using prefixes and suffixes such as: ace, aro, 'a', demi, grey, flux etc.).

- *What* type of attraction is concerned (using suffixes such as: sexual, romantic etc.).

Split attractions

An individual whose romantic and sexual attraction align (regarding 'who' or 'how' attraction is experienced) is called 'perioriented'. It is unnecessary to state both matching orientations in which a person is perioriented; for example: a *pansexual panromantic* person need only go by 'pansexual' (since a matching romantic attraction is implied unless otherwise stated).

However, an individual whose romantic and sexual attraction do not align (regarding 'who' and 'how' attraction is experienced) is 'varioriented'. By viewing/approaching sexual and romantic attraction as two distinct categories (known as the Split Attraction Model— SAM), varioriented people are able to easier define and classify their (sexual and romantic) orientations.

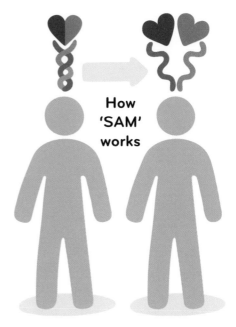

How 'SAM' works

The majority of varioriented people will be ace and/or aro (other than those who are specifically both asexual and aromantic—as this would be classed as perioriented). The SAM framework also provides a way for those who have allosexual and alloromantic orientations to distinguish non-aligned sexual and romantic attraction.

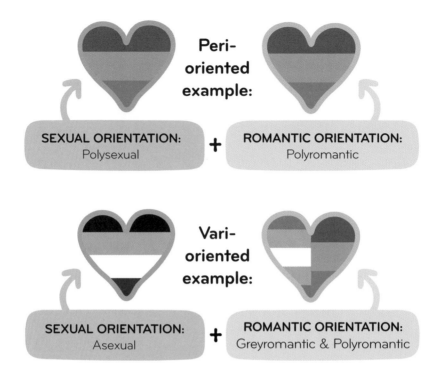

Peri-oriented example:

SEXUAL ORIENTATION: Polysexual **+** ROMANTIC ORIENTATION: Polyromantic

Vari-oriented example:

SEXUAL ORIENTATION: Asexual **+** ROMANTIC ORIENTATION: Greyromantic & Polyromantic

Acespec/alloromantic varioriented examples

Asexual and panromantic: no sexual attraction, but romantic attraction is experienced towards any gender.

Greysexual and biromantic: partial/limited/ambiguous sexual attraction is experienced, and romantic attraction is experienced to 'same/aligned and different' genders.

Demisexual lesbian and polyromantic: sexual attraction is experienced to women/non-men under very specific circumstances, and romantic attraction is experienced towards many (but not all) genders.

Arospec/allosexual varioriented examples

Aromantic and pansexual: no romantic attraction is experienced, but sexual attraction is experienced towards any gender.

Greyromantic and bisexual: partial/limited/ambiguous romantic attraction is experienced, and sexual attraction is experienced towards multiple genders.

Demiromantic lesbian and polysexual: romantic attraction may only be experienced to women/non-men under very specific circumstances, and sexual attraction is experienced towards many (but not all) genders.

Acespec/arospec varioriented examples

Asexual and greyromantic: no sexual attraction is experienced, but limited/partial/ambiguous romantic attraction is experienced.

Greysexual and demiromantic: limited/partial/ambiguous sexual attraction is experienced, and romantic attraction may only be experienced under very specific circumstances.

Demisexual and aromantic: sexual attraction may only be experienced under very specific circumstances, but no romantic attraction is experienced.

Allosexual/alloromantic varioriented examples

Polysexual and homoromantic: sexual attraction is experienced to many (but not all) genders, and romantic attraction is experienced towards those of the same/aligned gender.

Pansexual and heteroromantic: sexual attraction is experienced to all genders, and romantic attraction is experienced towards those of a different gender.

Homosexual and biromantic: sexual attraction is experienced towards those of the same/aligned gender, and romantic attraction is experienced towards multiple genders.

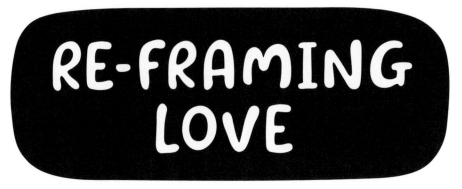

RE-FRAMING LOVE

EXPLORING HOW WE DEFINE FORMS OF LOVE

When we hear the word 'love', chances are, many people's first association will be with 'romantic love'. Societal and familial expectations often perpetuate a hierarchical view of love, in which romantic love ranks above all others. This can be seen via the 'compulsory alloromanticism' (the pressure/expectation to feel romantic attraction) and 'performative romance' (the pressure/expectation to want/engage in romantic actions) often expected within society.

By re-framing the narrative in which society determines the 'hierarchical value' of each form of love, it is, instead, the individual who actually defines it (e.g. according to the breadth/intensity to which it's experienced). For example, where one person might perceive and/or experience the love for their romantic partner (e.g. romantic love) as the most

fulfilling and significant form, another may perceive and/or experience the love for their child (paternal love) to be of equal (or perhaps higher) personal value.

Harmful love

In its extreme, any form of love can be considered harmful/unhealthy—due to its intensity and/or its effect on those involved. Regardless of whether or not love (in any form) is returned, it's helpful to remember that love should never be forced, be coerced, be assumed, or impact those involved in a consistently negative or damaging way.

These harmful manifestations may occur simultaneously, so, by understanding—and acknowledging—the differences between harmful/unhealthy experiences, help and support may be sought early on (from friends, family, qualified psychologists etc.).

Harmful/unhealthy manifestations of love can include:

 Manic love: a frenzied and/or intense experience in which the individual feels caught up in the experience. Manic love can be a common experience, but it becomes unhealthy when the individual's mental wellbeing and/or ability to function in daily life is consistently and negatively impacted.

 Obsessive love: an unhealthy focus/expectation is experienced towards the target.

 Possessive love: centres around the need for control; often connected to feelings of jealousy, perceived inadequacy, and/or a lack of trust.

 Unrequited love: a common and mostly harmless experience that usually dissipates on its own. Unrequited love can, however, become problematic when the desire/wants of the individual begin to severely impact their mental health, and/or when the target of their desire begins to feels threatened/unsafe.

Forms of love

Ancient Greek philosophers considered there to be many types of distinctive love, including:

- Philia: affectionate love (a platonic bond without any romantic feelings).

- Pragma: enduring love (affection that continues to grow/remain over time).

- Storge: familial love (a devoted emotional connection, such as between parent and child).

- Eros: romantic love (a desire for romantic affection and intimacy).

- Ludus: playful love (a flirtatious or light-hearted experience).

- Mania: obsessive love (a possessive, all-consuming experience).

- Philautia: self-love (an experience of self-worth/compassion).

- Agape: selfless love (an empathetic compassion for others).

A further way to define the different forms love can be to split the types into five common categories: parental, familial, romantic, alterous, and platonic.

Parental love: a selfless, enduring, and unconditional kind of love experienced by a parent (or parent-like figure) towards their child (or someone perceived as such).

Parental love might often include: philia, storge, and agape.

Familial love: a strong, affectionate bond experienced between those who are considered family. This bond can be with biological, adopted, or 'found/chosen' families, and can also include pets.

Familial love might often include: philia and storge.

Romantic love: this is the most difficult form of love to definitively define (since romance itself is a socio-cultural construction). One might consider romantic love to be an intense and intimate sense of affection between partners (or potential partners) in which typical/traditional romance-coded actions/feelings/expectations further this bond.

Romantic love might often include: ludus, eros, and pragma.

Alterous love: a form of love that could be considered as sitting somewhere between platonic and romantic, with a sense of both... though not enough to be clearly defined as either.

Alterous love might often include: ludus, philia, and pragma.

Platonic love: very similar to familial love, platonic love focuses on emotion, affection, and self-love. This bond is usually experienced between friends (in which it can also overlap with a sense of familial love) and/or those within a queerplatonic relationship.

Platonic love might often include: philia, storge, and philautia.

NOTE: Some of these forms are likely to overlap (platonic and familial, parental and familial etc.), while others specifically should not (e.g. parental and romantic) and specifically do not (e.g. platonic and romantic).

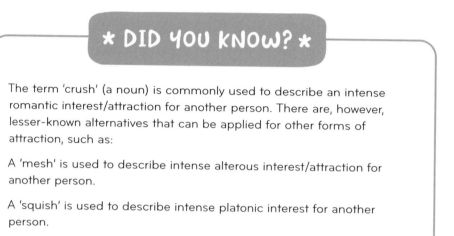

⭐ DID YOU KNOW? ⭐

The term 'crush' (a noun) is commonly used to describe an intense romantic interest/attraction for another person. There are, however, lesser-known alternatives that can be applied for other forms of attraction, such as:

A 'mesh' is used to describe intense alterous interest/attraction for another person.

A 'squish' is used to describe intense platonic interest for another person.

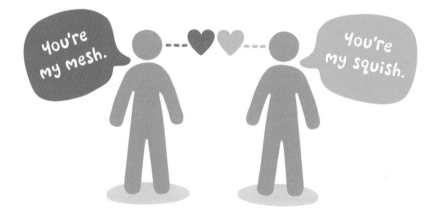

FIND YOUR FORM OF LOVE!

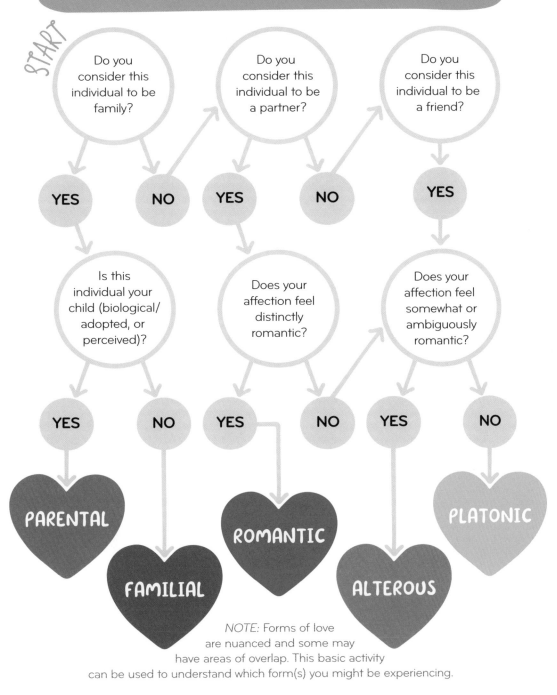

NOTE: Forms of love are nuanced and some may have areas of overlap. This basic activity can be used to understand which form(s) you might be experiencing.

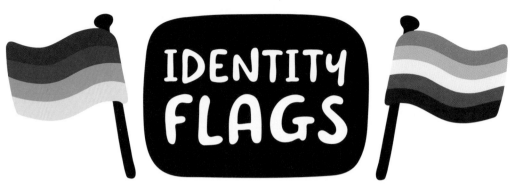

IDENTITY FLAGS

IDENTITIES WITHIN THE
ACE AND ARO COMMUNITIES

New flags and identities are continuously forming and evolving. Here, we explore some of the more established identities along with their flags.

* DID YOU KNOW? *

Microlabels are subcategories that describe an experience in more narrowed-down terms. An individual who identifies with a microlabel will also connect with a 'non-microlabel' from the relevant spectrum (e.g. an individual who feels a connection to the apothisexual microlabel may identify as asexual, and an individual who feels a connection to the cupioromantic microlabel may identify as greyromantic).

ACE**SPEC**

ARO**SPEC**

While it's common to see the asexual flag (black-grey-white-purple) representing the broad umbrella of asexual identities, it's also used for the specific identity: asexual.

The acespec flag (navy-purple-pink-cream/light pink) was posted on Tumblr in 2020 intended for use as an all-encompassing 'umbrella/spectrum' flag, rather than a flag for one specific identity.

Likewise, it's common to see the aromantic flag (green-green-white-grey-black) representing the broad umbrella of asexual identities, while also being used for the specific identity: aromantic.

The arospec flag (green-light green-cream-teal-dark teal/green), like the acespec flag, was also posted on Tumblr in 2020 to encompass the aromantic spectrum/umbrella.

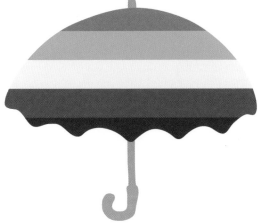

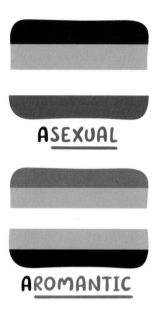

ASEXUAL

An orientation in which a person specifically experiences no sexual attraction. Beyond their orientation, an asexual person may experience other forms of attraction (aesthetic, romantic etc.) and can also have any level of libido.

AROMANTIC

A romantic orientation in which the individual specifically experiences no romantic attraction. An aromantic person may experience many forms of love/attraction, though none are experienced romantically.

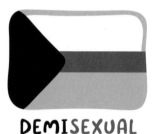

DEMISEXUAL

An experience in which distinct sexual attraction may occur for another person only once a strong emotional bond has formed. There is no guarantee as to when/if this feeling could occur.

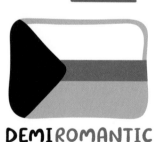

DEMIROMANTIC

An experience in which distinct romantic attraction may occur for another person only once a strong emotional bond has formed. There is no guarantee as to when/if this feeling could occur.

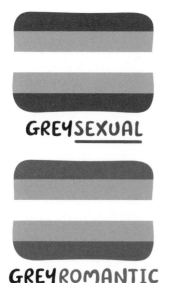

GREYSEXUAL

An identity and umbrella term. Sexual attraction may be experienced rarely (e.g. once in a lifetime), and/or weakly (e.g. not strong enough to act on), and/or ambiguously (e.g. uncertain if sexual attraction is experienced).

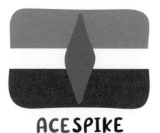

GREYROMANTIC

An identity and umbrella term. Romantic attraction may be experienced rarely (e.g. once in a lifetime), and/or weakly (e.g. not strong enough to act on), and/or ambiguously (e.g. uncertain if romantic attraction is experienced).

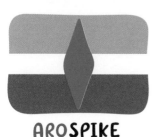

ACESPIKE

An identity in which a person feels mostly asexual (where no sexual attraction is experienced), but may experience spikes of sexual attraction for brief/indeterminate periods of time.

AROSPIKE

An identity in which a person feels mostly aromantic (where no romantic attraction is experienced), but may experience spikes of romantic attraction for brief/indeterminate periods of time.

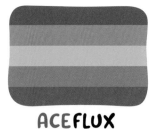

ACEFLUX

An identity that fluctuates between any of the orientations in the asexual spectrum (e.g. asexual, then demisexual, then greysexual—including the microlabels under the greysexual umbrella).

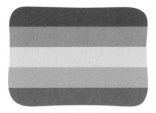

AROFLUX

An identity that fluctuates between any of the orientations in the aromantic spectrum (e.g. aromantic, then demiromantic, then greyromantic—including the microlabels under the greyromantic umbrella).

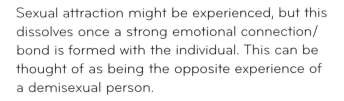

FRAYSEXUAL

Sexual attraction might be experienced, but this dissolves once a strong emotional connection/bond is formed with the individual. This can be thought of as being the opposite experience of a demisexual person.

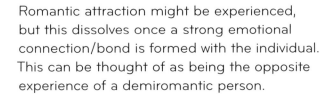

FRAYROMANTIC

Romantic attraction might be experienced, but this dissolves once a strong emotional connection/bond is formed with the individual. This can be thought of as being the opposite experience of a demiromantic person.

LITHOSEXUAL

Also known as akoisexual, sexual attraction may be experienced, but knowing it's reciprocated feels unwanted, causing any previous attraction experienced to dissipate. Different from fraysexual in that emotional connection does not play a part in the loss of attraction.

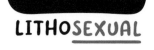

LITHOROMANTIC

Also known as akoiromantic, romantic attraction may be experienced, but knowing it's reciprocated feels unwanted, causing any previous attraction experienced to dissipate. Different from frayromantic in that emotional connection does not play a part in the loss of attraction.

FICTOSEXUAL

Used as an identity and umbrella term for individuals who experience little to no sexual attraction to others, but who do experience sexual attraction for fictional characters.

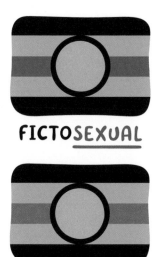

FICTOROMANTIC

Used as an identity and umbrella term for individuals who experience little to no romantic attraction to others, but who do experience romantic attraction for fictional characters.

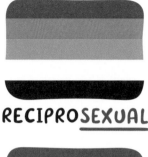

RECIPROSEXUAL

An experience in which sexual attraction may only occur once the individual knows the other person feels sexual attraction for them. There is no guarantee as to when/if this reciprocated feeling could occur.

RECIPROROMANTIC

An experience in which romantic attraction may only occur once the individual knows the other person feels romantic attraction for them. There is no guarantee as to when/if this reciprocated feeling could occur.

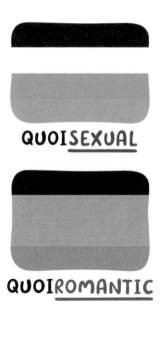

QUOISEXUAL

The suffix 'quoi' (pronounced 'kwah') comes from the French word meaning 'what'. Quoisexual people find themselves confused by, or disconnected from, the concept of sexuality and sexual attraction. The identity is also comically dubbed WTFsexual.

QUOIROMANTIC

Quoiromantic people find themselves confused by, or disconnected from, the concept of romanticism and romantic attraction. The identity is also comically dubbed WTFromantic.

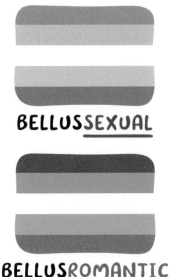

BELLUSSEXUAL

Bellussexual describes an experience in which the individual has an interest in certain sexual aspects/aesthetics or actions, yet do not, themselves, desire a sexual relationship (in addition to feeling little to no sexual attraction). (Microlabel)

BELLUSROMANTIC

Bellusromantic describes an experience in which the individual has an interest in certain romantic aspects/aesthetics or actions, yet do not, themselves, desire a romantic relationship (in addition to feeling little to no romantic attraction). (Microlabel)

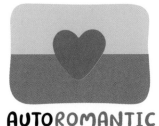

AUTOSEXUAL

An individual who experiences little to no sexual attraction and arousal to others, but does experience sexual attraction and/or arousal towards themselves.

AUTOROMANTIC

An individual who experiences little to no romantic attraction to others, but does experience romantic attraction towards themselves.

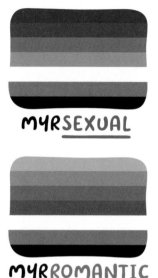

MYRSEXUAL

Multiple acespec orientations are experienced at the same time, with this identity feeling either static (e.g. consistently asexual and aegosexual) or fluctuating across the asexual spectrum (e.g. greysexual and fraysexual, shifting to asexual and aegosexual, and so on).

MYRROMANTIC

Multiple arospec orientations are experienced at the same time, with this identity feeling either static (e.g. consistently aromantic and aegoromantic) or fluctuating across the aromantic spectrum (e.g. greyromantic and frayromantic, shifting to aromantic and aegoromantic, and so on).

CUPIOSEXUAL

The individual specifically desires a sexual relationship simultaneously while little to no sexual attraction is felt. (Microlabel)

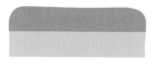

CUPIOROMANTIC

The individual specifically desires a romantic relationship simultaneously while little to no romantic attraction is felt. (Microlabel)

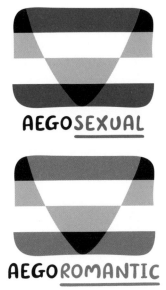

AEGOSEXUAL

Little to no sexual attraction is experienced, and while arousal can be experienced from sexual content or fantasies, this is experienced in a distinctly disconnected or omnipresent way (e.g. the individual might not imagine themselves engaging within the content). (Microlabel)

AEGOROMANTIC

Little to no romantic attraction is experienced, and while romantic feelings can be experienced from romantic content or fantasies, this is experienced in a distinctly disconnected or omnipresent way (e.g. the individual might not imagine themselves engaging within the content). (Microlabel)

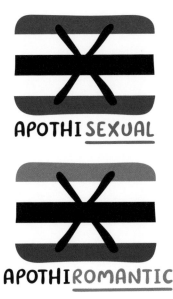

APOTHI SEXUAL

On the asexual spectrum, and specifically repulsed by the idea of sexual activity involving themselves. This may, or may not, extend to sexual content or sexual activity not involving themselves. (Microlabel)

APOTHIROMANTIC

On the aromantic spectrum, and specifically repulsed by the idea of romantic activity involving themselves. This may, or may not, extend to romantic content or activity not involving themselves. (Microlabel)

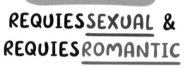

REQUIESSEXUAL &
REQUIESROMANTIC

Requiessexual can be used by those who feel unable to experience sexual attraction caused by some form of emotional exhaustion surrounding sex.

Similarly, requiesromantic can be used by those who feel unable to experience romantic attraction caused by some form of emotional exhaustion surrounding romance/romantic relationships.

Both identities are often connected to an individual's unique experience of neurodivergence or disability. (Microlabels)

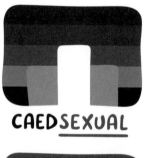

CAEDSEXUAL

Caedsexual is a label used by those who were able to experience sexual attraction in an allosexual way, yet are no longer able due to some form of emotional/physical trauma surrounding sex. (Microlabel)

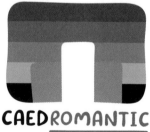

CAEDROMANTIC

Caedromantic is a label used by those who were able to experience romantic attraction in an alloromantic way, yet are no longer able due to some form of emotional trauma surrounding romance/romantic relationships. (Microlabel)

✶ DID YOU KNOW? ✶

People who connect with the requies-sexual/romantic and/or caed-sexual/ romantic microlabels have a specific cause for their ace/aro experience, so might be better considered as having an identity in which the experience of asexuality or aromanticism occurs (rather than an innate orientation).

AROACE

A combined sexual and romantic orientation (and umbrella term) in which the individual is anywhere on the aromantic spectrum and anywhere on the asexual spectrum (e.g. demiromantic and asexual).

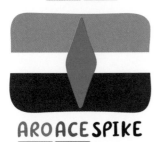

AROACESPIKE

An orientation in which the individual is both arospike and acespike, feeling mostly asexual and aromantic experiencing spikes of sexual and romantic attraction (not necessarily at the same time).

AROACEFLUX

An orientation in which the individual is both aroflux and aceflux, fluctuating across both the aromantic spectrum and the asexual spectrum.

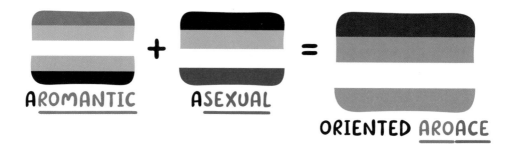

AROMANTIC + **ASEXUAL** = **ORIENTED AROACE**

An identity under the aroace umbrella in which the individual is specifically aromantic and asexual. An oriented aroace individual can experience significant forms of tertiary attraction (such as alterous, platonic, aesthetic, sensual, emotional etc.) alongside their aromantic and asexual orientations.

Examples may include: aromantic, asexual, and pan-aesthetic/sensual (pan-oriented aroace), or aromantic, asexual, and bi-queerplatonic (bi-oriented aroace).

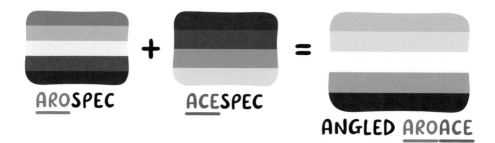

AROSPEC + **ACESPEC** = **ANGLED AROACE**

Under the aroace umbrella, angled aroace individuals are not strictly aromantic and asexual, experiencing significant, additional forms of romantic and/or sexual and/or tertiary attraction alongside their arospec and acespec orientations.

Examples may include: aromantic and demisexual/pansexual or aroflux/bialterous and demisexual/bisexual.

TRACE YOUR ACE IDENTITY!

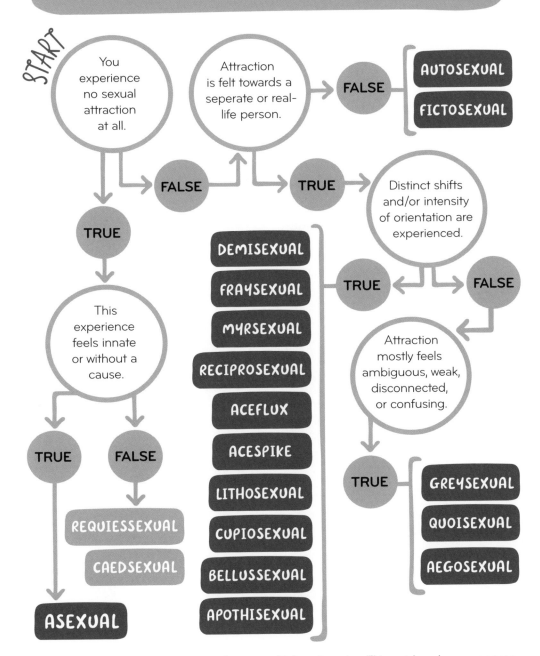

NOTE: Identities may overlap or fit into multiple categories. This guide only covers some of the basic elements used to define and/or narrow down different acespec identities.

NARROW YOUR ARO IDENTITY!

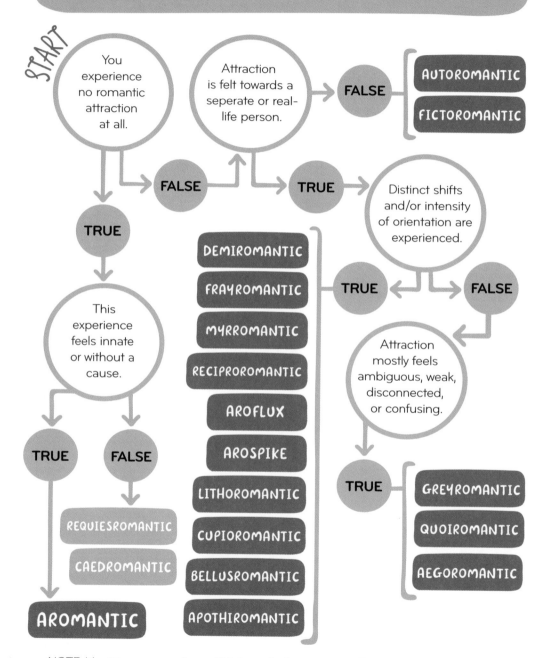

START

You experience no romantic attraction at all.

Attraction is felt towards a seperate or real-life person.

FALSE → AUTOROMANTIC / FICTOROMANTIC

FALSE → **TRUE** → Distinct shifts and/or intensity of orientation are experienced.

TRUE

This experience feels innate or without a cause.

DEMIROMANTIC
FRAYROMANTIC
MYRROMANTIC
RECIPROROMANTIC
AROFLUX
AROSPIKE
LITHOROMANTIC
CUPIOROMANTIC
BELLUSROMANTIC
APOTHIROMANTIC

TRUE ← / → **FALSE**

Attraction mostly feels ambiguous, weak, disconnected, or confusing.

TRUE → GREYROMANTIC / QUOIROMANTIC / AEGOROMANTIC

TRUE / **FALSE**

REQUIESROMANTIC
CAEDROMANTIC

AROMANTIC

NOTE: Identities may overlap or fit into multiple categories. This guide only covers some of the basic elements used to define and/or narrow down different arospec identities.

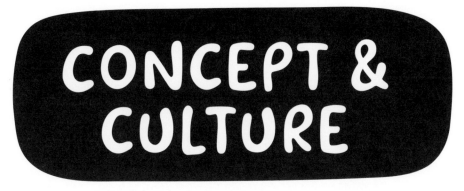

CONCEPT & CULTURE

THE PROGRESSION AND REPRESENTATION OF ASEXUALITY AND AROMANTICISM

The concept of asexuality

The term 'asexual' might feel relatively new among current-day LGBTQ+ terminology. In fact, a written concept of people who do not experience sexual desire (using terms such as 'monosexual' and 'anesthesia sexual') can be found from the mid to late 1800s.

An often-referred acknowledgement of asexuality can be found in Alfred Kinsey's publications *Sexual Behaviour in the Human Male* (1948) and *Sexual Behaviour in the Human Female* (1953). The introduced 'Kinsey scale' demonstrates the vast possibility of sexuality/sexual identities between those who identify as exclusively heterosexual and those identifying as exclusively homosexual. Among the rating scale of 0–6, an 'X' was used to represent those interviewed with no sexual desire or attractions.

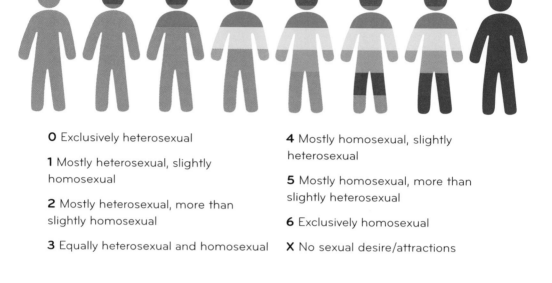

0 Exclusively heterosexual

1 Mostly heterosexual, slightly homosexual

2 Mostly heterosexual, more than slightly homosexual

3 Equally heterosexual and homosexual

4 Mostly homosexual, slightly heterosexual

5 Mostly homosexual, more than slightly heterosexual

6 Exclusively homosexual

X No sexual desire/attractions

Various publications continued to explore the concept/experience of asexuality throughout the mid to late 1900s, such as:

- The acceptance of asexuals (among heterosexuals, homosexuals, and bisexuals) mentioned in *The Satanic Bible* (1969) by Anton Szandor LaVey.

- Michael D. Storms revised the Kinsey scale framework within *Advances in the Study of Affect* (1979) to account for asexuality, expanding the original definition from no experience, to little to no experience of homoeroticism or heteroeroticism.

- An article written by Paula S. Nurius (titled 'Mental health implications of sexual orientation') in *The Journal of Sex Research* (1983), where asexuality was included and a distinction is made between sexual attitudes, activities, and attraction, and where: 'Individuals are categorised as either predominantly heterosexual, homosexual, bisexual, or asexual in their preferred sexual orientation.'[5]

- A 1997 StarNet Dispatches webzine article, 'My life as an amoeba', by Zoe O'Reilly, shone a light on the existence of asexuality and the lived asexual experience, stating: 'We want a colored ribbon, a national holiday, coupons for fast food. We want the world to know that we are out there.'[6]

Asexual representation

From the 2000s, the concept of 'asexuality' began to gain a little more traction. The world's largest online acespec community and information resource—the Asexual Visibility and Education Network (AVEN)—was created in 2001 by David Jay, through which the AVEN community selected the 2010 asexual pride flag design.

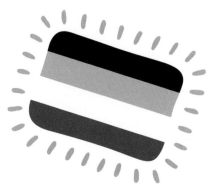

Between some of the sensationalised/harmful media portrayals of asexuality (e.g. Series 8, Episode 9, 2012, *House M.D.* 'Better Half' features an asexual-identifying character having their orientation 'disproven' as a medical condition) and possible 'queerbaiting' (the implication of queer representation within film/fiction, without any canonical confirmation) we do find some positive representation (most notably, Todd Chavez, in the Netflix animated series *BoJack Horseman*).

Fictional characters begin to be labelled as acespec by their creators, such as SpongeBob SquarePants (in Stephen Hillenburg's animated series of the same name) or Reyna Avila Ramírez-Arellano (from

---

5 Nurius, P.S. (1983) 'Mental health implications of sexual orientation.' *The Journal of Sex Research 19*(2), 119–136. Available at: www.jstor.org/stable/3812493, p.119.
6 https://web.archive.org/web/19970626042139/http://dispatches.azstarnet.com/zoe/amoeba.htm

Rick Riordan's *The Trials of Apollo* book series), and we start to see a rise in openly acespec people sharing ace/aro education or their 'lived experience' on social media (Yasmin Benoit, Rowan Ellis, Cody Daigle-Orians etc.).

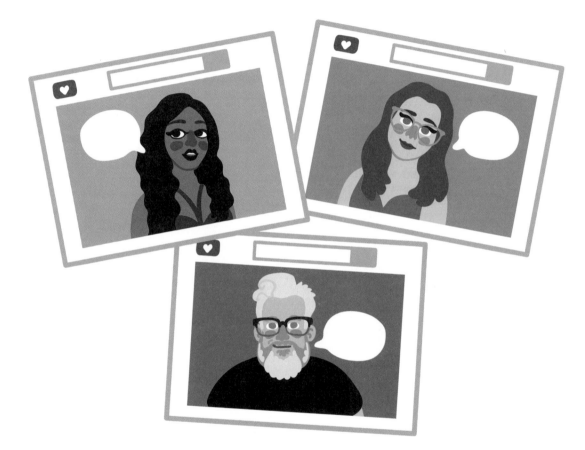

However, the distinct and commonplace inclusion of acespec identities/information (whether in fiction, non-fiction, media, or within sexual and relationship education) continues to remain minimal and infrequent. It is for this reason a normalisation and increased awareness of asexuality can highlight an often overlooked and invalidated minority group.

Positive examples of acespec representation can include:

- Education (or portrayals) based on accurate information and voices of the acespec community.

- Representation that shows the broad spectrum of acespec experiences and orientations.

- Asexuality that is not rationalised by a character's non-human status (robot, alien etc.).

- Asexuality that is not presented as a medical or mental health condition.

- Depictions where acespec orientations are clearly and distinctly confirmed within the content.

- Characters that aren't driven solely (or predominantly) by sexual attraction or sex.

The concept of aromanticism

'Aromantic' might be a relatively new term (appearing around 2002 on the Yahoo group Haven for the Human Amoeba), but the concept of 'aromanticism' (like asexuality) will have been experienced by people throughout history. The conflation or combination of romantic attraction and sexual attraction makes it particularly hard to source early written examples that specifically address alloromantic attraction (and the possible experience outside it).

Dorothy Tennov coined the term 'limerence' to articulate a profound sense of infatuation that can be experienced towards another person in *Love and Limerence: The Experience of Being in Love* (1979). Limerence often (but not exclusively) centres round romantic attraction, so Tennov's description of people as limerent and non-limerent can be viewed as: those who do experience intense romantic love, and those who do not experience intense romantic love (a possible indication that these people might have an arospec experience).

Aromantic representation

As aromanticism becomes further and more distinctly defined from asexuality, a similar path of awareness and representation (if a little slower) can be seen between the two spectrums. The aromantic pride flag was designed in 2014, while the Aromantic-spectrum Union for Recognition, Education and Advocacy (AUREA) was created in 2019 as an aromantic counterpart to AVEN.

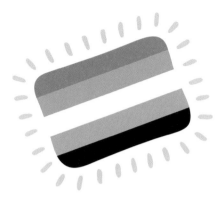

The few canonically confirmed arospec characters (such as Georgia from Alice Oseman's book *Loveless*, or Felicity Montague from Mackenzi Lee's 2018 book *The Lady's Guide to Petticoats and Piracy*) can be seen predominantly within fiction. Additionally, few public figures have confirmed their identity on the aromantic spectrum (without an additional acespec identity)—whether due to lack of arospec awareness or smaller community numbers... time will tell.

Examples of positive arospec representation to look out for include:

- Education (or portrayals) based on accurate information and listening to the voices of arospec people.

- A representation of the broad spectrum of arospec experiences and orientations.

- Aromanticism that is not rationalised by a character's non-human status (robot, alien etc.).

- Aromanticism that is not presented as a medical or mental health condition.

- Depictions where arospec orientations are clearly and distinctly confirmed within the content.

- Characters who aren't driven solely (or predominantly) by romantic attraction and romantic expectations.

Book recommendations

Why not investigate some inclusive fictional representation with ace/aro characters and/or themes:

- *Beyond the Black Door* by A.M. Strickland
- *Dare Mighty Things* by Heather Kaczynski
- *Elatsoe* by Darcie Little Badger
- *Every Heart a Doorway* by Seanan McGuire
- *Full Disclosure* by Camryn Garrett
- *Let's Talk About Love* by Claire Kann
- *Little Thieves* by Margaret Owen
- *Loveless* by Alice Oseman
- *Radio Silence* by Alice Oseman
- *Sawkill Girls* by Claire Legrand
- *Summer Bird Blue* by Akemi Dawn Bowman
- *Summer of Salt* by Katrina Leno
- *Tarnished Are the Stars* by Rosiee Thor
- *Tash Hearts Tolstoy* by Kathryn Ormsbee
- *The Lady's Guide to Petticoats and Piracy* by Mackenzi Lee
- *The Romantic Agenda* by Claire Kann
- *The Summer of Bitter and Sweet* by Jen Ferguson
- *Upside Down* by N.R. Walker

Culture

There are many unofficial objects, mascots, or symbols associated with (or representing) the ace and aro communities—diverse as the spectrums themselves.

These objects, mascots, or symbols are a playful way to explore some of the community-created associations. These can change over time, and will certainly vary according to an individual's opinion/exposure to them.

Ace culture

Black ring

An official acespec symbol is a black ring worn on a person's middle finger of their right hand. This is worn as a sign to other aces, and as a way to feel more connected to the ace community.

Purple

Inspired by many of the acespec flags, shades of purple are often used to promote, support, and embody ace-ness!

Dragons and axolotls

The dragon was adopted—in part—to combat those who view asexuality as something 'made up'. Hence, the ace mascot might as well be a *badass* mythical ('made-up') creature.

Because many people also seem to view asexuality as 'unusual'...well, here comes a cute, 'unusual' axolotl mascot to represent that!

Garlic bread and cake

This is commonly used in ace-related memes to humorously imply that garlic bread and cake are preferable to sex. It can also be common to see virtual cake (emojis or images) used to welcome new members of ace-related groups online.

Space ace

The common consensus of the term 'space ace' is that it generally reflects an ace person who loves all things outer space–related...in rhyming fashion!

Ace playing cards

It's in the name! The ace of spades symbol is most commonly used due to its recognisability.

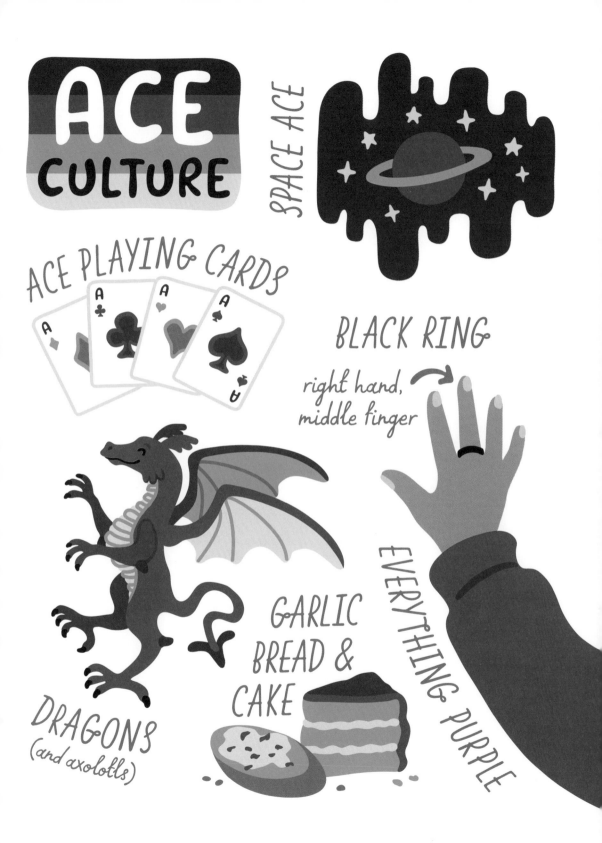

ACE CULTURE

SPACE ACE

ACE PLAYING CARDS

BLACK RING

right hand, middle finger

DRAGONS
(and axolotls)

GARLIC BREAD & CAKE

EVERYTHING PURPLE

Aro culture

White ring

An official arospec symbol is a white ring worn on a person's middle finger of their left hand. This is worn as a sign to other aros, and as a way to feel more connected to the aro community.

Green

Inspired by many of the arospec flags, shades of green are often used to promote, support, and embody aro-ness!

Griffins

As yet, no particular animal is consistently used by the aro community for their unofficial mascot. Griffins can sometimes be seen as a counterpart to 'ace dragons' (for similar reasons), along with suggestions including (but by no means limited to) tigers/cats, snakes, frogs, or praying mantises.

Herbs and plants

Plants are commonly connected to aro culture due to their green-hued nature—particularly herbs due to the 'aro-matic' pun connection. Yellow flowers can also be used to represent platonic love/friendship.

Aro-space

A pun on the word 'aerospace', this is used as a similar equivalent to 'space ace'.

Arrows and archery

Due to the similar pronunciation to the word 'aro', arrow symbols and archery are often used to represent aromanticism.

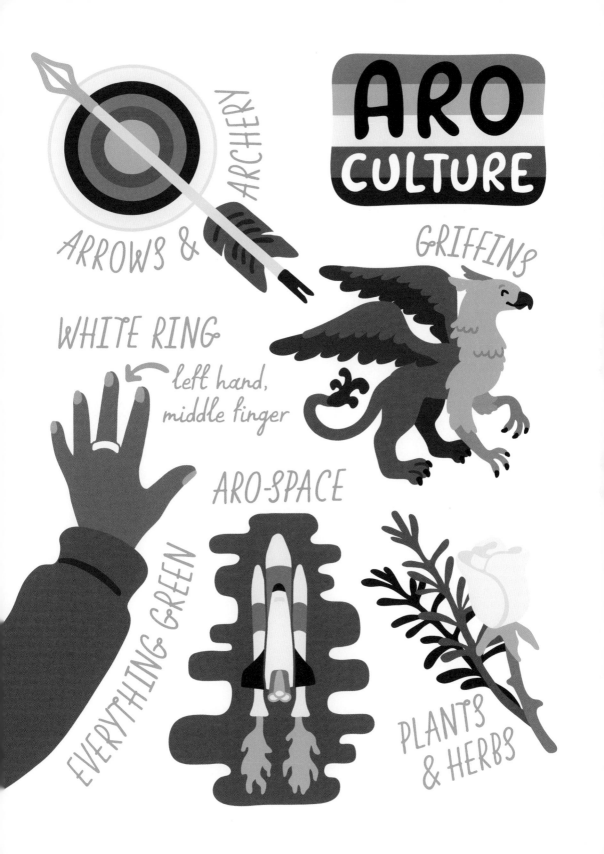

ARROWS & ARCHERY

ARO CULTURE

GRIFFINS

WHITE RING
left hand, middle finger

ARO-SPACE

EVERYTHING GREEN

PLANTS & HERBS

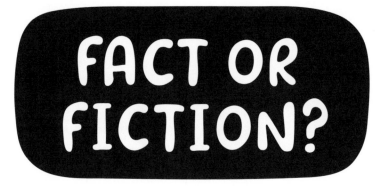

FACT OR FICTION?

ASSESSING ACE AND ARO ASSUMPTIONS

Things aren't always as *straight*forward as they seem when it comes to commonly held views about the asexual and aromantic spectrums. In this chapter we'll sort the fact ('true' statements) from the fiction ('false' statements).

Let's AROde some ACEsumptions!

'Acespec orientations can be fixed/cured'

False: An acespec orientation is natural, the same as any other sexual orientation; it is neither a mental nor a medical disorder. Examples of innate asexuality could include:

- An individual who has always felt little to no sexual attraction (regardless of libido, and with no specific cause for this experience).

- An individual who learns about asexuality later in life, realising they fall on the asexual spectrum.

- An individual who finds their sexual orientation is (or has become) fluid/changeable, shifting into the asexual spectrum (regardless of libido, and with no specific cause for this experience).

Some people will experience little to no sexual attraction from a specific cause (e.g. from mental ill health or trauma), and this might be better defined as an 'experience of asexuality' rather than an 'acespec orientation'. In these instances, professional treatment to address mental health/trauma would likely be beneficial/recommended (particularly where an experience of asexuality causes personal distress).

'Sexual attraction is the same as libido'

False: Sexual attraction is aimed towards someone, an innate desire to engage in sexual activity with a specific person. Libido can occur

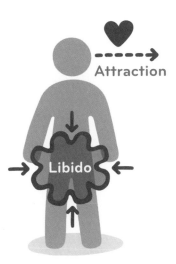

alongside sexual attraction, but these are two separate experiences. Libido itself is not directed towards anyone; it is an aroused state with a desire for sexual release (caused by fluctuating hormones, physical stimulation etc.).

A person's sexual orientation is only defined by sexual attraction—the gender(s) it's experienced towards and/or how it's experienced (asexuality and allosexuality)—never how high or how low their libido is.

'Being acespec is the same as being celibate'

False: Acespec orientations are defined by how an individual innately experiences sexual attraction. Celibacy is a specific choice not to engage in sexual activity (whether the individual experiences sexual attraction or not).

'Acespec people don't have sex'

True and False: Some acespec people do, but others don't. This is because *innate feelings* (i.e., sexual attraction), *choices* (i.e., a decision to participate in sexual activity), and *actions* (i.e., actively engaging in sexual activity) are three separate things. An individual can make the choice to participate in sexual activity, and then actively engage in sexual activity, all without needing to experience any innate feelings of sexual attraction. Some may choose to do so (for their partner, to sate their libido etc.), or because they do experience some partial/limited/circumstantial feelings of sexual attraction.

'Acespec people don't masturbate'

True and False: Simply put, some ace folks do, and some don't. It's a preference for each individual if/why they make the choice to do so.

'Acespec people don't feel romantic love'

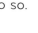

True and False: Many will confuse asexuality with aromanticism, or automatically assume that an ace person will also be aro. While some ace folks also reside on the aromantic spectrum, this is not the default. Many people with an acespec orientation will have a romantic orientation that does not reside on the aromantic spectrum (such as being ace and biromantic).

'Arospec orientations can be fixed/cured'

False: An arospec orientation is natural, the same as any other romantic orientation; it is neither a mental nor a medical disorder. Examples of innate aromanticism can include:

- An individual who has always felt little to no romantic attraction (with no specific cause for this experience).

- An individual who learns about aromanticism later in life, realising they fall on the romantic spectrum.

- An individual who finds their romantic orientation is (or has become) fluid/changeable, shifting into the aromantic spectrum (with no specific cause for this experience).

Some people will experience little to no romantic attraction from a specific cause (e.g. from mental ill health or trauma), and this might be better defined as an 'experience of aromanticism' rather than an 'arospec orientation'. In these instances, professional treatment to address an individual's mental health/trauma would likely be beneficial/recommended (particularly where an experience of aromanticism causes personal distress).

'Being arospec is the same as being picky'

False: Arospec orientations are defined by how an individual innately experiences romantic attraction, while being critical ('picky') about potential romantic partners centres around thought and reasoning.

'Arospec people don't exhibit romantic behaviour'

True and False: Innate feelings (i.e., romantic attraction), choices (i.e., the decision to participate in romantic behaviour), and actions (i.e., actively engaging in romantic behaviour) are three separate things.

So, an acespec individual might choose to participate in romantic behaviour, and then actively engage in romantic behaviour without needing to experience any innate feelings of romantic attraction. Some may do so for their partner, or because they experience some partial/limited/circumstantial feelings of romantic attraction.

'Being arospec means a fear of commitment'

False: A fear of commitment (known as 'gamophobia') is a phobic disorder. There is a difference between an innate experience of little to no romantic attraction and the act/decision of commitment.

'Being arospec means an inability to love'

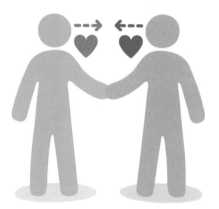

False: This assumes 'romantic love' as the only form of love a person can experience. Some arospec orientations may experience a partial/limited/circumstantial form of romantic love, but having an arospec orientation does not mean lacking the ability to experience love of any kind.

Arospec individuals might love deeply in ways such as platonic, alterous, familial, or parental.

'Arospec people don't want relationships'

True and False: Concerning partnered relationships, some arospec individuals may choose/desire to be in a fully/somewhat romance-coded relationship while others will not.

Arospec people may also desire a committed *queerplatonic relationship* (known as a QPR—entirely platonic-based), a polyamorous relationship, or even a 'soft romo' relationship (based on a low level of romance-coded behaviours).

ACEPHOBIA & AROPHOBIA

RECOGNISING PREJUDICE AND DISCRIMINATION

The definition of 'phobia'

Aside from its application to describe an intense or irrational fear of something, 'phobia' can also mean an intense dislike of or aversion to something. In the same way the term 'homophobia' can be used to describe an intense dislike of or aversion to gay and lesbian people (their existence, relationships etc.), *acephobia* and *arophobia* can be applied when the same/similar phobic attitudes/responses are directed at people as a direct result of their ace or aro identity.

Ace/arophobic attitudes and discrimination

Content warning: Mentions of violence, sexual coercion, rape, and suicidal ideation.

Prejudice

Negative/untrue/hostile opinions (often preconceived and/or automatic) about a particular group of people. For instance, assuming all arospec people are heartless and must use their identity as an excuse to 'sleep around' would be a prejudiced and unfounded opinion.

Erasure

A refusal to believe or acknowledge acespec or arospec identities, and/or a failing of (or disregard of) ace and aro representation, awareness, and educational content. For example, in a worldwide survey, where the majority of participants were aged between 14 and 24, 95% of acespec people reported a lack of asexual inclusion within sex education or discussion topics at school, with only 2% first hearing about asexuality via school.[7]

Dehumanisation

Assuming/insisting there be a reason for an individual's identity. Arospec people often endure the assumption they have an inability to feel emotion, any form of love, or empathy; they are viewed as inhuman, robotic, or even psychopathic, while acespec people are often presumed defective in that their sexuality must have a mental or physical cause.

Until the fifth edition of the *Diagnostic and Statistical Manual of Mental Disorders* (DSM-5, 2013), an individual with an acespec orientation would have met the diagnostic criteria of hypoactive sexual desire disorder (HSDD). Currently, a diagnosis of a sexual interest/arousal disorder is not to be made if an individual self-identifies as asexual (or acespec). While technically distancing acespec orientations from that of a mental/physical disorder, the DSM-5 can still be problematic for those unable to self-identify due to a lack of awareness about the spectrum, risking not only an inaccurate diagnosis but also unnecessary treatment.

Harassment and violence

It's not too difficult to find LGBTQ+ people who have experienced

---

7   Weis, R., Hermann, L., Bauer, C., *et al.* (2021) *2019 Ace Community Survey Summary Report*. The Ace Community Survey Team, pp.33, 34.

sexual harassment, coercion and/or violence—including acespec and arospec people. This can be backed by the 2020 Ace Community Survey Summary Report data,[8] showing 40.6% of ace people receiving attempts or suggestions from others to 'fix/cure' their identity. Page 72 of the same report reveals 59.1% of acespec respondents experiencing some form of 'contact sexual violence' (of which, 53.6% accounted for unwanted sexual contact, 26.2% for sexual coercion, and 18.8% for rape).

Pressure to conform

Society is structured around the compliance and continuation of heteronormative, allonormative, and amatonormative behaviours. In navigating a world where these ingrained expectations surrounding sex, romance, and relationships seem rigidly set, those who do not conform (such as acespec and arospec people) may have a higher risk of mental ill health. Indeed, reports indicate a correlation, with 39.8% of acespec people who've experienced a lack of identity-affirming healthcare also experiencing suicidal ideation in the past 12 months. Furthermore, similar percentages were found linking other factors, such as attempts at 'fixing' an acespec person's orientation, or the experience of verbal or sexual harassment.[9]

Further evidence

In 2012, Cara MacInnis and Gordon Hodson published a paper, 'Intergroup bias toward "Group X": Evidence of prejudice, dehumanisation, avoidance, and discrimination against asexuals',[10] to explore the possibility of acephobic attitudes. Results confirmed

8 Hermann, L., Baba, A., Montagner, D., *et al.* (2022) *2020 Ace Community Survey Summary Report*. The Ace Community Survey Team. Available at: https://acecommunitysurvey.org, p.93.
9 Ibid, p.91.
10 MacInnis, C.C. and Hodson, G. (2012) 'Intergroup bias toward "Group X": Evidence of prejudice, dehumanization, avoidance, and discrimination against asexuals.' *Group Processes & Intergroup Relations* 15, 6. Available at: https://doi.org/10.1177/1368430212442419

heterosexual participants as displaying a higher rate of negative and dehumanising attitudes towards asexuals than to other queer minority groups.

The UK 2018 National LGBT Survey Research Report also holds some interesting asexual-based results:[11]

- Asexuals both scored low on life satisfaction[12] and were found to feel the least comfortable being LGBTQ+ in the UK when measured against the other orientations included.[13]

- 89% of the asexual-identifying respondents also avoided an openness about being LGBTQ+ in their daily lives for fear of a negative reaction from others.[14]

- Asexual people reported similar rates to gay and lesbian people when asked about sexual harassment or violence (from those they do not live with), with 1.5% of asexuals and 1.6% of gay/lesbians reporting the experience.[15]

- Asexuals also reported the second highest percentage[16] of all identities included that were offered conversion/reparative therapy to 'cure' them of being LGBTQ+ (with trans men rating over 9% and asexuals at 8%).

NOTE: Aromanticism, unfortunately, is vastly understudied, so reliable statistical data was unavailable for this section.

11 Government Equalities Office (2018) *National LGBT Survey, Research Report, July 2018.* Manchester. Available at: https://assets.publishing.service.gov.uk/government/uploads/system/uploads/attachment_data/file/721704/LGBT-survey-research-report.pdf
12 Ibid, p.28.
13 Ibid, p.31.
14 Ibid, p.47.
15 Ibid, p.68.
16 Ibid, p.85.

ACE-PHOBIC BINGO!

MARK COMMENTS YOU'VE HEARD ABOUT BEING ACE.

'You need to speak to a doctor.'	'You need to speak to a psychologist.'	'There must be something wrong with you!'	'You don't suffer discrimination, so you're not LGBTQ+.'
'Well you're unattractive, so no one cares.'	'But you're so attractive... what a waste!'	'You just can't get laid.'	'Spend a night with me... that'll fix you.'
'You'll change your mind when you meet the right person.'	'You'll change your mind when you're older.'	'You can't be ace if you have sex or masturbate.'	'How do you know unless you've tried having sex?'
'If you have a sex-positive attitude you're not ace!'	'You must be a prude.'	'That goes against human nature!'	'You're depriving your partner of sex!'
'But you don't dress/seem ace.'	'If you're into BDSM/kink you're not ace!'	'That's just another word for celibacy.'	'If you have a libido then you're not ace.'

NOTE: This page features a combination of common acespec micro-aggressions, general discriminatory attitudes (ranging in severity), and some LGBTQ+ ignorance/misinformation.

ARO-PHOBIC BINGO!

MARK COMMENTS YOU'VE HEARD ABOUT BEING ARO.

'That's not a real thing.'	'You need to speak to a psychologist.'	'There must be something wrong with you!'	'You don't suffer discrimination, so you're not LGBTQ+.'
'You must be so sad/lonely!'	'You'll eventually find someone to love you.'	'You're just being picky.'	'Love takes work. You just need to try harder.'
'You'll change your mind when you meet the right person.'	'You'll change your mind when you're older.'	'Your life must be so unfulfilled!'	'How do you know if you've never been in love?'
'If you have a romance-positive attitude you're not aro!'	'You must be a psychopath.'	'That goes against human nature!'	'You're depriving your partner of love!'
'But you don't behave/seem like you're aro.'	'If you want to be (or are) married then you're not aro!'	'You just have a fear of commitment.'	'If you have/had crushes then you're not aro.'

NOTE: This page features a combination of common arospec micro-aggressions, general discriminatory attitudes (ranging in severity), and some LGBTQ+ ignorance/misinformation.

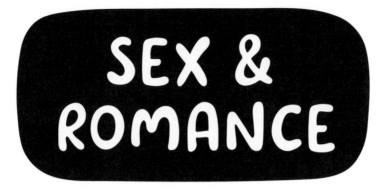

UNDERSTANDING VIEWS, COMFORT LEVELS, AND BOUNDARIES

Views on sex and romance

There are different ways for an individual to distinguish their feelings about personally engaging in/with sexual and/or romantic activity or content, which are not to be confused with an individual's attitude toward sex or romance in a broader sense.

Any combination of these feelings and attitudes can be experienced and may not necessarily align as expected (e.g. an arospec individual may personally feel 'romance repulsed' but hold a general 'romance neutral' attitude).

Personal feelings

How an individual feels about personally engaging in/with sexual and/or romantic activity or content can either remain 'fixed' (non-shifting) or feel as though it fluctuates (due to circumstance or orientation).

Sex repulsed: feeling repulsed by the idea of engaging in/with sexual activity, thoughts, or content.

 Sex averse: not wanting to engage in/with sexual activity or content.

 Sex indifferent: no strong feelings (either way) about engaging in/with sexual activity or content.

 Sex favourable: feeling comfort/desire/inclination about engaging in/with sexual activity or content.

 Romance repulsed: feeling repulsed by the idea of engaging in/with romantic activity, thoughts, or content.

 Romance averse: not wanting to engage in/with romantic activity or content.

 Romance indifferent: no strong feelings (either way) about engaging in/with romantic activity or content.

 Romance favourable: feeling comfort/desire/inclination about engaging in/with romantic activity or content.

General attitude

This attitude relates to the general idea/expression/action of sexual and/or romantic activity or content that does not personally involve oneself. These broader attitudes may be more likely to remain 'fixed' (non-shifting):

Sex positive: having an open/progressive attitude towards sex and sexual aspects.

Sex neutral: having a neutral/disinterested attitude towards sex and sexual aspects.

Sex negative: having a closed/intolerant attitude towards sex and sexual aspects.

Romance positive: having an open/progressive attitude towards romance and romantic aspects.

Romance neutral: having a neutral/disinterested attitude towards romance and romantic aspects.

Romance negative: having a closed/intolerant attitude towards romance and romantic aspects.

★ DID YOU KNOW? ★

According to the 2019 Ace Community Survey Summary Report,[17] 45% of aces were sex repulsed or averse, 42% were indifferent or uncertain, 9% were sex favourable, and 4% considered their experience as fluctuating/other.

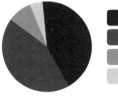

- ■ Sex repulsed or averse
- ■ Sex indifferent or uncertain
- ■ Sex favourable
- ■ Fluctuating/other experience

17 Weis, R., Hermann, L., Bauer, C., *et al.* (2021) *The 2019 Ace Community Survey Summary Report*. The Ace Community Survey Team, p.59.

Types of sexual and/or romantic relationships

To define/classify relationship types it can be helpful to understand what sexual or romantic attraction may be experienced within it (by one or more of the participants).

TYPE OF CHOSEN RELATION-SHIP ↓	Often involves attraction that's:			May involve attraction that's:		
	Romantic	Sexual	Alterous	Romantic	Sexual	Alterous
Romantic	*				*	*
Sexual		*		*		*
Alterous			*	*	*	
Soft Romo				*	*	*

Relationship boundaries and comfort levels

It's important, within any relationship type, to regularly (and honestly) assess and communicate the comfort levels and boundaries for each participant involved (since levels may drastically change or fluctuate depending on circumstances, partner, or environment etc.).

Created primarily (but not exclusively) with aro and ace individuals in mind, the worksheets that follow can be used to examine (some) personal boundaries and comfort levels for sexual or romantic/alterous/soft romo relationships.

COMFORT LEVELS & BOUNDARIES

(For 'romantic', 'alterous', or 'soft romo' relationships)

What is your romantic orientation (e.g. panromantic)?	
Personal romantic feelings (romantic aspects or activities, specifically involving oneself)	Repulsed ☐ Indifferent ☐ Averse ☐ Favourable ☐
General romantic attitude (view of romance and romanticism beyond oneself)	Negative ☐ Positive ☐ Neutral ☐

CONSENSUAL ASPECT OR ACTIVITY	Yes	Some-times	Maybe	Unsure	No
Taking part in typically romantic dates					
Chaste kissing (forehead, closed mouth, cheek etc.)					
Brief affectionate touch (hands/face, hugging etc.)					
Extended affectionate touch (hand holding, cuddling etc.)					
Eye gazing (intimate and/or prolonged)					

CONSENSUAL ASPECT OR ACTIVITY	Yes	Some-times	Maybe	Unsure	No
Are you comfortable saying 'I love you'?					
Are you comfortable being told 'I love you'?					
Being referred to as a 'boyfriend' or 'girlfriend'					
Being referred to as a 'partner'					
Celebrating or acknowledging Valentine's Day					
Celebrating or acknowledging relationship anniversaries					
Having a 'closed' romantic relationship (monogamy)					
Having an 'open' romantic relationship (polyamory)					

Any additional concerns or preferences:

COMFORT LEVELS & BOUNDARIES

(For 'sexual' relationships)

What is your sexual orientation (e.g. pan-demisexual)?	
Personal feelings about sex (sexual aspects or activities, specifically involving oneself)	Repulsed ☐ Indifferent ☐ Averse ☐ Favourable ☐
General attitude about sex (view of sex and sexuality beyond oneself)	Negative ☐ Positive ☐ Neutral ☐

CONSENSUAL ASPECT OR ACTIVITY	Yes	Some-times	Maybe	Unsure	No
Heavy kissing (open mouth, tongues etc.)					
Consuming sexual content with your significant other					
Being partially naked in front of your significant other					
Being fully naked in front of your significant other					
Over-the-clothes touching (groping, frottage etc.)					

CONSENSUAL ASPECT OR ACTIVITY	Yes	Some-times	Maybe	Unsure	No
Masturbation in front of your SO					
Watching your SO masturbate					
Using non-penetrative sex toys on your SO—GIVING					
Having non-penetrative sex toys used on you—RECEIVING					
Using penetrative sex toys on your SO—GIVING					
Having penetrative sex toys used on you—RECEIVING					
Pleasuring your SO with your hands—GIVING					
Your SO pleasuring you with their hands—RECEIVING					
Having oral sex with your SO—GIVING					
Having oral sex with your SO—RECEIVING					

NOTE: 'SO' refers to 'significant other' (or sexual partner)

CONSENSUAL ASPECT OR ACTIVITY	Yes	Some-times	Maybe	Unsure	No
Having non-penetrative sex (e.g. intercrural)—GIVING					
Having non-penetrative sex (e.g. intercrural)—RECEIVING					
Having penetrative sex with your SO—GIVING					
Having penetrative sex with your SO—RECEIVING					
Having a 'closed' sexual relationship (monogamy)					
Having an 'open' sexual relationship (polyamory)					

Any additional concerns or preferences:

NOTE: 'SO' refers to 'significant other' (or sexual partner)

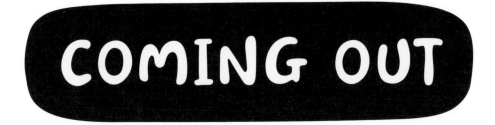

COMING OUT

CONSIDERING THE WHY, WHEN, HOW, WHERE, AND TO WHOM

Why?

Reasons for coming out can include: freedom of self-expression, being able to openly live as your queer authentic self, not having to hide aspects of your identity/life, or a sense of readiness (emotional and mental).

Reasons for not coming out (yet, or at all) can include: being in an unsafe environment/home life/workplace; fear/expectation of bullying, harassment, or violence; not feeling ready; personal privacy; or that it feels unimportant/unnecessary.

When?

There is no age or time limit to when an individual can 'come out'... and you don't ever need to 'come out' if that feels personally right for you. You might choose to do so when you're able to articulate what your identity means to you, or simply when you feel comfortable with your identity.

How and where?

You can choose whichever method of communication feels

most comfortable or safe, whether this is in-person, a public announcement (online), via phone/text, or even in a letter. For safety, ensure you are able to readily exit any location you choose for in-person communication.

Who?

It can be preferable to ensure those you come out to are trustworthy: friends, family, colleagues/students, therapists/mentors etc. If you wish for only a few specific people to know, be sure to tell them this (to avoid others finding out).

Navigating reactions

Positive reactions

The person/people you come out to may have questions about your identity and your experience of it. It's not your responsibility to educate the people in your life about your identity, but it can be especially helpful to provide a list of useful

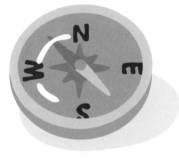

information resources. If you are happy to provide answers, that's great too...just remember, you are under no obligation to answer highly personal/probing questions if it makes you feel uncomfortable.

Negative reactions

There is the possibility of a negative reaction after coming out. This might present as disbelief, hostility, harassment, or even violence.

For harassment problems online, you might want to block/report users or adjust profile settings to 'private'. If you feel threatened or unsafe (in-person) immediately try to remove yourself from the location/perpetrator. Try to report any threats, harassment, or violence (whether at home, place of work/education etc.) to a trusted individual (or the relevant authorities).

In addition, remember to be vigilant of your mental health. If you feel you're struggling, speak to trained mental health professionals, contact free mental health/LGBT+ helplines, or try reaching out to the queer community for support.

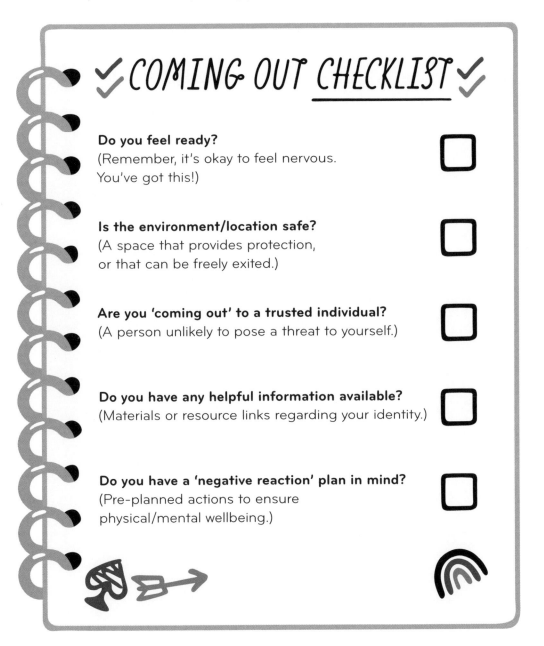

✓ COMING OUT CHECKLIST ✓

Do you feel ready?
(Remember, it's okay to feel nervous.
You've got this!) ☐

Is the environment/location safe?
(A space that provides protection,
or that can be freely exited.) ☐

Are you 'coming out' to a trusted individual?
(A person unlikely to pose a threat to yourself.) ☐

Do you have any helpful information available?
(Materials or resource links regarding your identity.) ☐

Do you have a 'negative reaction' plan in mind?
(Pre-planned actions to ensure
physical/mental wellbeing.) ☐

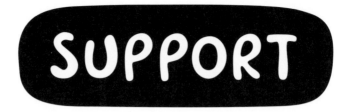

SUPPORT

A LIST OF RESOURCES, DATES, AND INSPIRATION

Ace and aro resources

LGBTQ+ wellbeing

- The Trevor Project, www.thetrevorproject.org: The Trevor Project is the world's largest suicide prevention and crisis intervention organisation for LGBTQ+ youth. If you or someone you know needs help or support, The Trevor Project's trained crisis counsellors are available 24/7 at 1-866-488-7386, via chat at TheTrevorProject.org/Get-Help, or by texting START to 678678.

- Galop, https://galop.org.uk: A UK helpline service for LGBTQ+ people affected by violence and abuse. LGBT+ Domestic Abuse Helpline: 0800 999 5428, LGBT+ Conversion Therapy Helpline: 0800 130 3335, LGBT+ Hate Crime Helpline: 020 7704 2040.

- Switchboard LGBT+ (UK) Helpline, https://switchboard.lgbt: A safe space for anyone to discuss anything, including sexuality, gender identity, sexual health and emotional wellbeing. Call: 0300 330 0630 (10am–10pm daily) or email: chris@switchboard.lgbt

- 988 Suicide & Crisis Lifeline, 988lifeline.org/help-yourself/lgbtq: For confidential support with 24/7 crisis counsellors call/text 988, or chat online via the website.

Acespec

- AVEN (The Asexual Visibility & Education Network), www. asexuality.org: The world's largest online asexual community, including a large archive of resources on asexuality.

- Asexuals.net, www.asexuals.net: A (paid membership) dating website for acespec people looking for love or friendship.

Arospec

- AUREA (Aromantic-spectrum Union for Recognition, Education, and Advocacy), www.aromanticism.org: A volunteer-based initiative—developing the best resource for aromantic-spectrum people.

- Arocalypse, www.arocalypse.com: A discussion forum for all arospec identities.

Acespec and arospec

- Aces & Aros, https://acesandaros.org: A hub for ace and aro people to get involved in their community.

Ace and aro celebrations

Some internationally recognised days/weeks celebrating asexuality and aromanticism:

Ace Week

Usually held around the last week in October, with specific dates varying from year to year. Find out more at: https://aceweek.org

International Asexuality Day (IAD)

Currently set each year on 6 April. Find out more at: https://internationalasexualityday.org

Aromantic Spectrum Awareness Week

Usually held in late February, with specific dates varying from year to year. Find out more at: www.arospecweek.org

Online tags

Across various platforms (Instagram, Twitter, Tumblr, TikTok etc.), you could search using the hashtags:

- #ace #asexual #asexuality #ascespec #asexualspectrum
- #aro #aromantic #arospec #aromanticspectrum
- #aroace #aromanticasexual

For memes and musings, check out the www.reddit.com subreddits:

- r/aromantic, r/aaaaaaaarrrrro, r/asexual, r/asexuality, r/ace, r/aaaaaaacccccccce, r/aromanticasexual, r/AroAceMemes

Ace and aro public figures

Plenty of speculation has been made about historical figures (such as Emily Brontë, or T.E. Lawrence), and even fictional characters (such as Sherlock Holmes) as to their place on the asexual and/or aromantic spectrum. It is, however, those who can apply current-day LGBTQ+ language to openly discuss their ace and aro orientations who make the greatest impact.

'Real-person' representation of ace and/or aro individuals existing openly can provide an incredible boost to normalise and demystify such orientations for people within and beyond the communities.

Here are some ace and/or aro public figures you might find interesting, helpful, or inspirational:

- Yasmin Benoit, she/her (www.yasminbenoit.co.uk): An asexual/aromantic model and activist. Creator of #ThisIsWhatAsexualLooksLike.

- David J. Bradley, he/they (www.youtube.com/c/DavidJBradley): An aro/ace creator of video essays, reviews, and aspec education.

- Angela Chen, she/her (www.angelachen.org): Asexual journalist, editor, and author of *ACE: What Asexuality Reveals About Desire, Society, and the Meaning of Sex*.

- Michaela Cole (https://twitter.com/michaelacoel): An aromantic BAFTA- and Emmy Award-winning actress, screenwriter, director, producer, and singer.

- Cody Daigle-Orians, he/they (https://acedadadvice.com): The asexual creator of 'Ace Dad Advice' (acespec education via social media) and author of *I Am Ace*.

- Rowen Ellis, she/her (www.rowanellis.com): Asexual lesbian, author of *Here and Queer*, and creator of queer-focused video essays on YouTube.

- Connie Glynn, she/they (connieglynn.com): Aromantic author of the pentalogy series *The Rosewood Chronicles*.

- Ashabi Owagboriaye, she/they (Instagram: @_aceingrace_): The creator of Ace In Grace, a space providing ace education with a spotlight on BIPOC representation and inclusion.

- David Jay: Asexual activist and founder of AVEN (The Asexual Visibility and Education Network).

- Alice Oseman, she/they (aliceoseman.com): Aroace creator of works such as *Radio Silence*, *Loveless*, and the million-copy bestselling *Heartstopper* series.

- Gabriel Picolo, he/him (www.instagram.com/_picolo): An ace comic book artist, illustrating DC Teen Titans graphic novels *Raven*, *Beast Boy*, and *Beast Boy Loves Raven*.

- Robin Skinner, he/they (www.youtube.com/user/fluffybluehat): An ace and aro musician, known professionally as Cavetown.

Disclaimer: These public figures have spoken (in some form) about their orientation/experience residing on the asexual and/or aromantic spectrum. Sexuality and romanticism can be fluid and changeable, so there is no guarantee any stated orientations will remain as such for the individuals mentioned.

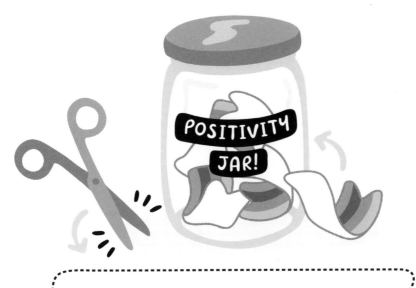

POSITIVITY JAR!

FILL A JAR WITH THE CUT-OUT SLIPS
AND USE FOR SOME POSITIVITY!

Love and intimacy take many forms
and are expressed in many ways.

It's okay to feel confused.
Take all the time you need.

It's okay if labels aren't
your thing.

We are all human.
We are all equal.

You are part of a wonderful
and diverse community!

Never feel guilty about being
your authentic queer self.

Queer rights are
human rights!

Society doesn't get to
decide your orientation.

Create and seek out
safe spaces.

It's okay if your orientation
shifts/changes over time.

Celebrate
diversity.

Valid, valid, valid,
valid, valid!

You are
not broken!

The human experience is better defined by
ethics and empathy, not sex/romance.

LGBTQ+ identities are
queer-ly natural!

ACKNOWLEDGEMENTS

I'd like to thank Jessica Kingsley Publishers and Hachette for helping to bring this idea to fruition; being so dear to my heart, I'm thrilled to be able to share this project with a wider audience!

Particular thanks are due to the wonderful Andrew James, who provided me with the courage and spark to further pursue my passion for queer education, along with the fantastic JKP team involved in this project, including Laura Dignum-Smith, Hannah Snetsinger, and Adam Peacock.

My biggest thanks go to every person (ace, aro, or ally) who supported me on my queer journey; to every person who shared their story, or thanks, or encouragement—I hope I can convey how truly grateful I am, because your words continue to inspire me to this day!

You are all incredibly *amazing*, and extremely *awesome*!

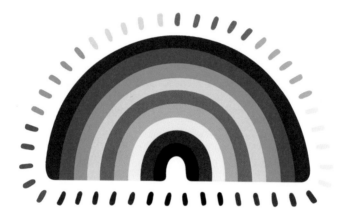

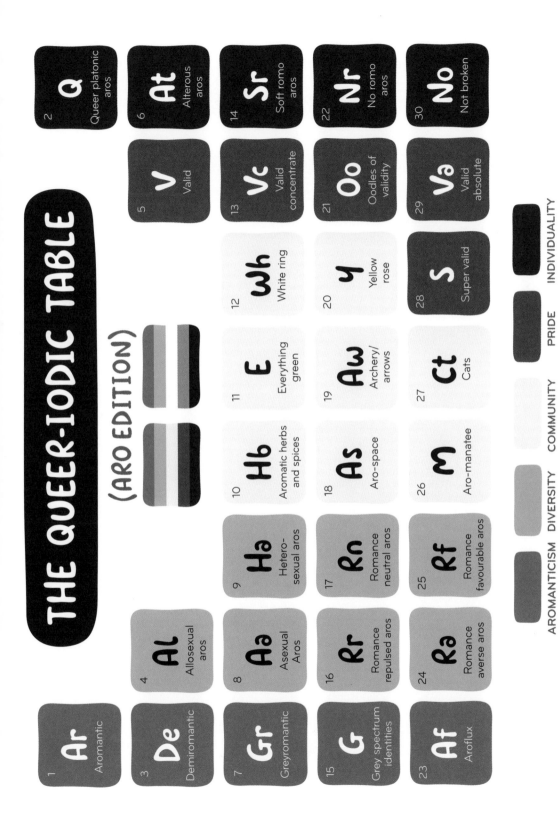

THE QUEER-IODIC TABLE

(ARO EDITION)

1 **Ar** Aromantic					2 **Q** Queer platonic aros
3 **De** Demiromantic	4 **Al** Allosexual aros			5 **V** Valid	6 **At** Alterous aros
7 **Gr** Greyromantic	8 **Aa** Asexual Aros	9 **Ha** Hetero-sexual aros	10 **Hb** Aromatic herbs and spices	11 **E** Everything green	12 **Wh** White ring	13 **Vc** Valid concentrate	14 **Sr** Soft romo aros
15 **G** Grey spectrum identities	16 **Rr** Romance repulsed aros	17 **Rn** Romance neutral aros	18 **As** Aro-space	19 **Aw** Archery/arrows	20 **Y** Yellow rose	21 **Oo** Oodles of validity	22 **Nr** No romo aros
23 **Af** Aroflux	24 **Ra** Romance averse aros	25 **Rf** Romance favourable aros	26 **M** Aro-manatee	27 **Ct** Cats	28 **S** Super valid	29 **Va** Valid absolute	30 **No** Not broken

AROMANTICISM **DIVERSITY** **COMMUNITY** **PRIDE** **INDIVIDUALITY**

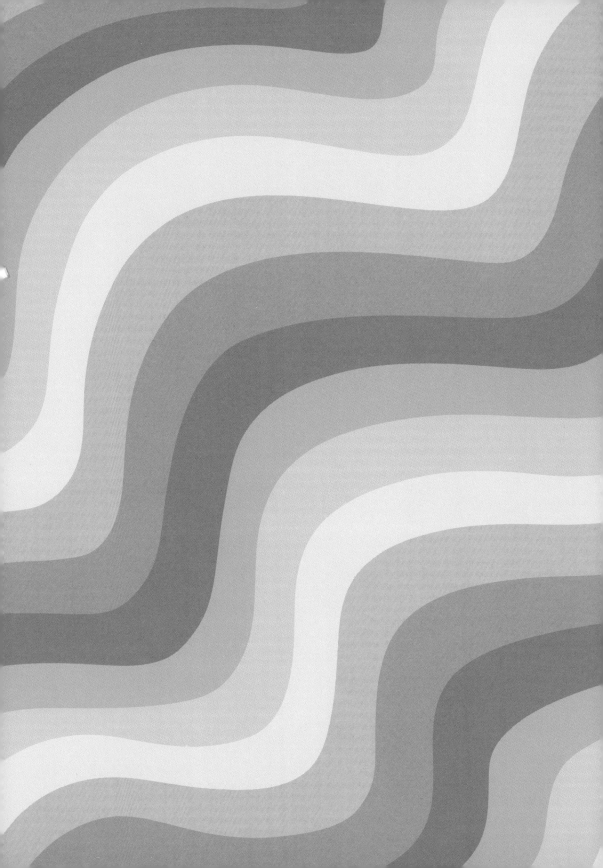